pilates

a *flowmotion*™ title

pilates

introduction by
suzanne scott

Sterling Publishing Co., Inc.
New York

Created and conceived by
Axis Publishing Limited
8c Accommodation Road
London NW11 8ED
www.axispublishing.co.uk

Creative Director: Siân Keogh
Managing Editor: Matthew Harvey
Project Designer: Zoë Dissell
Project Editor: Dr. Louise Aikman
Production Manager: Sue Bayliss
Photographer: Mike Good

Library of Congress Cataloging-in-Publication
Data Available

10 9 8 7 6 5 4 3 2 1

Published in 2002 by Sterling Publishing Co., Inc.
387 Park Avenue South, New York, NY 10016
Text and images © Axis Publishing Limited 2002
Distributed in Canada by Sterling Publishing
C/o Canadian Manda Group,
One Atlantic Avenue, Suite 105
Toronto, Ontario, M6K 3E7, Canada

Separation by United Graphics Pte Limited
Printed and bound by Star Standard (Pte) Limited

Sterling ISBN 0–8069–8873–8

a *flowmotion*™ title

pilates

contents

introduction

Although you may only recently have heard or read about Pilates, it has been in existence for about eighty years. Once dubbed "the fitness world's best kept secret," it remained relatively unknown because there were few instructors trained to teach it and even fewer studios with the equipment used for some of the exercises.

Over the last five years, the popularity of Pilates has grown beyond recognition, leading one writer to label it "the fastest growing global fitness trend."

You can now find Pilates matwork classes in most health clubs and public leisure centers and specialized studios are opening up independently in clubs and spas. You may be offered Pilates-style exercises by your health care practitioner if you have a back problem, or you may be doing some Pilates already in the "core stability" part of your usual fitness class at the gym.

So what is it?

To get the most out of your Pilates class, or if you are using this book and practicing at home, you need to understand a little about the background of the Pilates system and the principles behind it. Developed by Joseph Pilates (1880–1967), the Pilates method is an interrelated system of exercises designed to challenge your strength, flexibility, and coordination. Joseph Pilates firmly believed that fitness was not just about developing and maintaining perfect, muscular bodies and gaining fitness and competitive performance, but a "unity of mind, body, and spirit."

Perhaps it is this philosophy as well as the benefits of the exercises themselves that account for people converting to his system in such numbers.

When you perform a Pilates exercise you are never just tightening one area of the body, stretching another, or mindlessly powering your way through a series of reps.

Each movement requires your full concentration as you train yourself to control your alignment and target your body's deeper muscles. As part of the process, you also have to learn to let go of the muscle tension that distorts your posture and your ability to perform the exercises correctly. To help achieve this, a flowing breathing pattern has to be mastered for each exercise.

PILATES is a whole-body system that develops inner strength and flexibility—not just muscle size.

PRINCIPLES ARE PRINCIPLES....

In the years since his death, Joseph Pilates' original exercises have been developed by many teachers around the world, often making use of new knowledge that we have about how the body works and how to exercise effectively.

The following key principles still hold true, although each Pilates teacher has his or her own approach and may emphasize things a little differently depending on his or her experience and focus.

- **concentration**
- **control**
- **center**
- **alignment**
- **breathing**
- **flowing movement**

Understanding what each principle means will help you to get the most out of this book and your Pilates practice.

concentration and control

A famous quotation of Joseph Pilates reads "it is the mind that builds the body." Recent research seems to back this up. Using computer imaging, it is now possible to show that just thinking about moving a muscle sends a shower of impulses through the nervous system.

Pilates uses this "imaging" to get the most out of each movement. You have to be mindful not mindless when you do Pilates so, to help you, consider the following points before you begin:

- choose a time of day when you are least distracted or likely to be interrupted
- make sure the room is warm and that you have a comfortable mat to work on
- do not exercise if you have just eaten or are hungry— your concentration will be impaired
- if you choose to play music, pick something that will stay in the background without a strong beat
- whatever is bothering you—leave it behind. You will need all your attention for the exercises

Many Eastern systems believe this "one pointedness" is the key to self-development. Joseph Pilates was aware of this, but in building his own system, he focused on developing mental control by linking mind and body in a practical way, using breathing and visualization with each exercise. In a Pilates studio or class, the teacher will help you do this by using key words or images to give you the "visual flavor" or feel of the moves.

To help you do this at home, study the photographs and the text for each exercise and try to picture each movement in your mind's eye before you begin. Visualize yourself performing the moves in the pictures and imagine the feeling of the muscles you will be using as indicated in the text.

This "mental rehearsal" is important; it will help to get the correct muscles working (something a teacher would normally check for you by looking or feeling for muscle activity) and put a stop to others overworking. Bad posture and habits often cause muscles to work when they don't need to. Pilates encourages us to let go of old patterns so that new and better ones can take their place.

Joseph Pilates believed that movement should be controlled and subject to our will rather than our whim (or somebody else's). In typical fitness training, the "getting into" a move is often targeted more than the getting out. We pay attention as we load our muscles, but forget that how we unload them is just as important.

Pilates requires you to be aware of your body—how you are holding it, which muscles are about to be relaxed, and which are about to be activated—throughout each exercise.

Pilates stresses that the "eccentric" part of movement (returning to rest) is as important, perhaps even more important than the active, "concentric" part. When it comes to exercise, both need to be addressed.

This is why Pilates is often used as a key element in advanced fitness training or in rehabilitation programs after injury. Joseph Pilates seems to have predicted this, and you can benefit from his discoveries by paying attention to the following "technique" points:

● Practice how you get into and out of an exercise. For example, in a spine curl, how you curl out of the move is as crucial as how you curl up into it. Train your body not to slump or collapse out of an exercise, but return your spine to the mat or limbs back to the start position carefully.

● Practice an "arc of control"—give equal weight and attention to all parts of the exercise so you don't speed through the tougher parts. Your limbs are your levers, and you need to control their weight and direction of movement to gain the maximum benefit from the exercises.

center and alignment

This is perhaps the most important Pilates principle, and the one responsible for many of the benefits claimed for the method. For Joseph Pilates the center (or "powerhouse," as he called it) was to be activated throughout each exercise. Pilates teachers often talk about creating a strong center from which movement can flow. What they mean by this is focusing on core muscles around the spine, the lower abdominals and the pelvic floor to create a stable base for all movement.

Pilates himself advocated a bracing or pulling in of the abdominals. Most teachers now suggest a more gentle hollowing designed to target the deeper abdominals rather than the "six pack." The following exercise will help you achieve this. Try to practice it several times a day, first lying down and then sitting and standing.

Lying in relaxation position, place your hands on your lower abdomen. Breathe in gently, and as you breathe out, draw the lower part of your abdomen in toward your spine ("hollowing"). If your abdomen "kicks up" under your hands or bulges, you are working too hard—aim for a gentle tension like a drum skin being gradually tightened.

Use the breathing to help you (breathing out makes the hollowing or tightening easier to feel), and then practice holding the gentle contraction while you breathe quietly in and out. Now try this exercise standing and sitting. Once you master the basic abdominal contraction, you can put it into your Pilates exercising—ideally this "pre-activation" should happen at the start of each exercise and run on quietly in the background while your other muscles coordinate the movements.

NEUTRAL The abdominals have been hollowed. Engaging the muscles around the spine, the lower abs and pelvic floor helps control the back's position.

OVERARCHING Here, the shape and position of the back needs more abdominal work to bring it closer to "neutral". This position is unstable.

TUCKING UNDER Here, the neutral curve has been lost and the lower spine flattened into the mat. The spine is not in its natural position.

Pilates requires you to multi-task. As you work through an exercise, you have to think not only about the muscles you are working (and not working), but also your overall body position.

Your alignment refers not only to the placement of your spine and limbs in a given exercise, but also your posture in daily life. Good posture relies on a series of gentle curves in the spine. Pilates can help you to achieve better posture and restore the healthy spinal curves. For good alignment, there should be a long, shallow curve in the lower back (the "lordosis"). If your back arches too far from the mat, try padding under the tail of your spine with a folded towel.

If your back flattens into the mat, try placing a small rolled towel under your lower back so your spine curves gently away from the mat. Now check the position of your head—you may need to pad either under the neck or the back of your head to get a similarly gentle neck curve.

To check your standing posture, look front—and side-on in a mirror. Ideally, you should be symmetrical in the shoulders, rib cage, hips, knees, and ankles from the front, and the gentle curves should be visible from the side. Few of us have ideal posture, and it is best to think of it as a long-term aim that you can use Pilates to work toward. It is beyond the scope of this book to attempt individual correction—seek advice if you have problems related to your posture. Then use these exercises to help you work on improving posture with help from your Pilates teacher.

LOOKING in a mirror, the body should be symmetrical, limbs held evenly when at rest and joints level.

SIDE VIEW The spine should form gentle S curves. Exaggerated or flattened curves reveal poor posture.

breathing

The most difficult part of Pilates is usually the breathing. For each exercise you have to align, center, breathe, and move. Your pattern of breathing should flow with the exercise. Original Pilates had set patterns of breathing for each move. Most teachers nowadays use breathing to help the effect of each exercise and improve control of posture and alignment.

You can practice Pilates breathing in the relaxation position (below). Place your hands on either side of your rib cage, and as you inhale, try to breathe gently into your hands—you should feel your back widen slightly. As you breathe out, press lightly with your palms so the ribs close a little

and roll down slightly toward the waist. This is the side breath or lateral breathing used in Pilates. It helps to offset the tendency to tense the neck and shoulders in shallow breathing or abdominal breathing (when the stomach pushes out and in with each breath), which make it harder to center and use the deep abdominals correctly.

Try to follow the breathing cues in the book, as they are designed to work with each exercise. Practically, you may want to grade your learning —begin with centering, alignment, and mentally rehearsing the moves, adding the breathing once you have mastered this.

THE RELAXATION position, with knees bent, spine relaxed, and hands on the pelvis, is the best position for practicing lateral breathing. This will help you achieve much more effective exercising in your Pilates routine.

WORK ON your posture in a sitting position. As in standing, look for a gentle curve in the spine and watch for tucking or overarching, which can indicate poor posture and alignment.

EXTEND your legs and check your posture again. Different positions put different stresses on the spine. Working from the center to support good spinal curves is the key to correct alignment.

TO CHECK whether you are breathing laterally, hold your hands on your ribs under your armpits. Lateral breathing should cause the ribs to move sideways into your hands.

BREATHING can be used to enhance stretches and change the focus of exercises. If you lie with your hands above your head, you can feel the upper back arch up as you breathe in and the chest expands.

flowing movement

The Pilates system was intended as flowing movement, not statically held postures. Watching someone who is experienced at Pilates perform the exercises, you will be struck by their economy of movement and their controlled, graceful execution.

The unique format of the photographs in this book will help you reproduce this, as you can see how one movement flows into the next. Have this in mind as you mentally rehearse your Pilates and as you are performing the exercises. You should be aiming for a steady, flowing movement between each stage of an exercise, as illustrated by the images.

Joseph Pilates believed that his innovative exercise method was the best way to achieve both health and happiness. This is the goal of Pilates, and as with any effective system, it should become part of your daily routine. It takes dedicated practice to master this thoughtful, mindful technique, but the benefits to mind and body, experienced by thousands of users already, will reward all your efforts. Refer to the information on the opposite page before starting to use the *FlowMotion* Pilates sequences.

Suzanne Scott

USE FLOWMOTION to achieve a flowing movement throughout your exercises. Each stage of every movement is pictured.

go with the flow

The special *Flowmotion* images used in this book have been created to make sure that you see the whole of each exercise—not just selected highlights. Each exercise is labelled suitable for beginners, intermediate, or advanced students by a colored tab above the title. The captions along the bottom of the images provide additional information to help you perform the exercises confidently. Below this, another layer of information includes instructions for breathing and symbols indicating when to hold a position. The order the exercises are shown in the book is a suggested sequence only. Beginners should pick out suitable exercises, while intermediate and advanced exercisers can create their own programme.

beginners | intermediate

hip flexor stretch

rectus femoris, iliacus and adductors

hip flexor stretch | 45

As the name suggests, this routine focuses on stretching the muscles that cross the hip, encouraging greater hip mobility. Beginners should hold the pose of the first image and not add the upper body twist. Keep the lower abdominals hollowed throughout and use padding to the knee as required. This exercise is not suitable if you have knee, hip, or lower back problems.

● Start with your right knee stretched out behind you and your left knee bent with your hands resting upon it. Breathe in and lengthen your spine.

● Lunge forward, keeping the head upright. Contract your abdominals so as not to compress your lower back. Reach your arms out and begin to turn to the left. Reach toward the floor only as far as is comfortable.

● Circle the right arm up over the head and stretch your right leg straight, keeping it close to the floor. Place the palm of your left hand on the floor and turn your head to face toward it.

● Now, start to sit back onto your right leg as you bring your arm back over your head again. Keep your shoulders down as you move your arm and think "tall" into your spine keeping your abdominals drawn in.

● As you sit back on your right leg, your left leg should form a 90 degree angle to the floor. Bring your right arm back down to your right side.

● Looking forward again, bring both hands to rest on your left knee. Repeat this exercise, beginning with the left knee stretched out behind you.

inhale   exhale   inhale   exhale   inhale   exhale   inhale

■ This indicates the beginning or end of a sequence, where there is no movement.

▶ This indicates continued movement in the sequence.

‖ This indicates a pause, either to hold a pose, stretch or take a number of breaths.

turn outs core stability and adductor stretch

This is an excellent exercise to help increase flexibility in the hip joint by stretching your adductors. As it is such a gentle exercise, it can be practiced by those with limited flexibility and those who are new to Pilates. Focus on keeping the supporting leg still to challenge your core control.

● Lie on your back with your knees bent and your hands on your pelvis. Breathe in and lengthen the spine.

● Bring your right leg up to a 90 degree angle with the knee still bent. Then turn out the knee. Keep your back flat on the floor and your neck relaxed.

● Point your foot as you turn the knee. You should feel the stretch on your inner thigh.

● Bring the knee back down again and rest for a few moments with your hands on your pelvis. Keep your neck lengthened and your gaze toward the sky.

■   ‖ **begin to exhale**   ▶   **exhale**   ▶   **inhale**   ▶

● Then raise your left leg up, pointing the toes as you do so, and keeping the supporting leg still and steady. Keep your shoulders down and relaxed.

● Raise the leg up to a 90 degree angle and then turn the knee out as before. Again, make sure your lower back remains on the floor as you perform this stretch.

● Bring your left leg down to the floor again. Make sure you keep the movement slow, controlled, and precise.

● Finish this exercise in the same position as you started. Relax your whole body and breathe deeply.

begin to exhale ▶ exhale inhale ‖ ▶ ‖

knee drops *stability and adductor stretch*

This exercise is suitable for beginners and will help you develop pelvic stability ("core control").

Begin by dropping the knee only as far as you can while keeping the supporting knee and hip still.

As your stability improves, drop the leg further for a gentle stretch along the inner thighs (adductors).

● Start this exercise in the relaxed position with your feet flat on the floor, your back straight, and your hands on your pelvis. Breathe in and lengthen the spine.

● Start to drop your right leg outward toward the floor. Keep your left knee still and isolate the movement in your right hip as your knee drops.

● Slowly take the leg toward the floor. Be careful not to twist your back while you are performing this move. Keep both buttocks on the floor.

● Take the leg down to the floor or as far as is comfortable. Keep your spine and neck lengthened and then breathe in.

● As you breathe out, start to raise your right leg back up toward your other knee. Keep your elbows soft and your hands resting lightly on your pelvis.

● Bring your leg up so that it is parallel with the other knee. Make sure this is a slow and controlled movement and that you maintain the curve of your spine (neutral).

● When you have reached the starting position again, take a breath in, then as you breathe out, start to lower your left knee outward to the floor. Repeat the whole routine using your left leg.

● When you have finished this routine, lie in the relaxed position and take a few deep breaths before beginning the next exercise.

begin to exhale   ▶ **exhale**   **inhale**   **exhale ‖**   ▶   ‖

sliding arms and legs

This exercise helps to develop your "center". You should focus on keeping your pelvis and ribs still as your arms and legs work. Aim for flowing movements of your limbs as your abdominals draw in to support your spine and create your center.

● Start by lying on your back with your knees bent and your feet flat on the floor. Have your arms relaxed and resting on your stomach. Breathe in and lengthen the spine.

● Start to lower your right leg down toward the floor, keeping your left leg bent and your shoulders relaxed.

● Make sure your neck is lengthened and not tense. Slide the leg down to the floor without locking your knee. Flex, point, and slide it back up again. Repeat using the left leg.

● Put your left hand onto your right rib. Raise your right arm in the air. Point your fingers away from you and concentrate on isolating the movement in the arm so as to avoid hunching the shoulder.

II inhale   ▶   exhale   inhale   ▶   begin to exhale   ▶

● Bring your right arm back toward the floor. Keep your arm lengthened and make sure this is a slow and controlled movement.

● Extend your arm right over your head so it is aligned with the rest of your body. Keep your back flat on the floor and be careful not to let your neck become tense. Breathe in. Do not force your arm back.

● Bring the arm back down again toward your legs and rest it on your hip. Repeat this arm movement with your left arm.

● Finish the exercise in the starting position. Have both hands resting on your hips and your body relaxed and aligned.

exhale   ▶ inhale   exhale   ❙❙   ▶   ❙❙

knee and leg circles *and hip rotators*

This original Pilates exercise improves the pelvic stability and the mobility of the hip joint. Beginners should keep both legs bent at the knee throughout and use the stretch band for support. The leg circles demand a high level of core control and flexibility. Do not attempt them if you are a beginner. If you have lower back problems, seek medical advice before using any part of this exercise.

● Lie on your back with your knees bent and your arms by your side. Breathe in and lengthen the spine. Pick up your stretch band and place it under your left knee.

● Allow your leg to relax and drop slightly to the side. Don't move your legs, let the movement come from your hips. This loosens your hips and teaches you to move from the hip. Repeat with the other leg.

● Return your knees to the center and put the stretch band to one side. Have your arms by your side with the palms facing down. Raise your left leg up in the air and extend it as you reach.

● Now draw some wide semicircles in the air with your toes pointed. Remember to avoid arching your back and keep your neck relaxed.

‖ exhale ▶ inhale exhale ▶ exhale ▶

● Stretch the right leg out with the toes pointed. Keep it raised 1–2 inches (2–4 centimeters) above the floor and perform another semicircle in this position.

● Try to make the semicircle as wide as possible. However, do not force or strain your legs in any way. Keep your back flat on the floor and the rest of your body still.

● As you complete the semicircle concentrate on keeping your legs lengthened, but don't lock your knees.

● When you have finished this exercise, lower both legs to the floor and then repeat the whole routine with your right leg.

inhale   exhale   ▶ exhale   inhale   ‖   ▶   ‖

first connection

arm reach and biceps curl, *latissimus dorsi, biceps and deltoids*

This exercise works the major muscles of the upper back and arms. If you focus on the position of your shoulders, (don't hunch or pinch the shoulder blades together) it will help to develop stability in your shoulder girdle. Intermediate exercisers can use weights to add resistance.

- Begin the exercise in the standing position with your hands by your side. Keep your back lengthened and be careful not to arch it at any point in the stretch. Keep your shoulders relaxed and wide.

- Before beginning the exercise, breathe in, contract your abdominals, and lengthen the spine. Grip the weights securely with your palms facing back. Squeeze your arms into your body and feel the biceps relax.

- Breathe out as you move your arms slowly back. Concentrate on lengthening your arms as they move backward, as though you were reaching into the floor. Keep your elbows soft, your shoulders relaxed.

- As you begin to turn your hands around to come forward, take a breath in. Keep your eyes horizontal and focus on a spot directly ahead of you. Concentrate on keeping the back of the neck long and the head upright.

■   ▶ **inhale**   ▶ **exhale**   ▶ **inhale**   ▶

● Breathe out as the arms are extended all the way forward with your palms upright. Keep your spine straight and imagine that the tail of it is rooted into the ground.

● As you breathe in, begin to turn your hands around to face the ground and start to take your arms back to your sides again. Be careful not to let your weight move back. Breathe out as your arms go all the way back.

● Once the arms are back, take a deep breath in, then on the out breath, bring your arms forward again, bending your knees as you do. Bring your arms back to the side of your body.

● Now curl the forearms up, keeping the upper arms very still. As you raise your hands, keep your wrists straight and do not allow your elbows to drop. Breathe in as you release the arms and then relax.

exhale ▶ inhale exhale ▶ inhale exhale ▶ inhale   II

chest stretch

pectorals arm rotators and deltoids

This exercise strengthens the major muscles of the arms, shoulders, and upper back. Beginners should perform this without weights. People with shoulder problems should avoid the arm raise and only take the "offering" as far as is comfortable. Keep your head, neck, and shoulders aligned.

● Start with the arms bent at the elbows, holding the weights in the palms of the hand with the fingers pointing forward. Grip the weights with your thumbs. If you are not using weights, use the same hand position.

● Breathe in to prepare, checking that the spine is lengthened and the shoulders wide and relaxed. Start the chest stretch by moving the hands out from the body, keeping the elbows locked at your waist.

● Continue the stretch as far as you can—the ideal is for both lower arms to end up parallel with each other. Move the hands back to the center and then repeat the stretch four times.

● Now grip the weights and start to lower your arms, bending the elbows out as you go.

● When the weights are level with your pelvis, hold the position for a second and take a breath. Again, check that your spine is still lengthened and your shoulders are not hunched.

● As you breathe out, start to lift your arms up and out to the sides. As the hands rise, begin to turn them so the palms are facing forward.

● When your arms reach shoulder level, your palms should be facing forward. As you continue to reach up, keep rotating the hands until the palms are uppermost.

● Steadily bring the arms together above your head. They shouldn't touch, but should rest about fist width apart. Breathe in as you let your arms return to your sides. Repeat the arm raise four times.

begin to exhale ▶ ▶ ‖ inhale ▶

lateral raise and pec press

You may be familiar with these movements from working out in a gym. The arm sequence works the muscles at the front and back of the chest (pectorals, rhomboids and trapezius), and upper arm (deltoids). When you perform them with a Pilates focus, keep your spine aligned and your lower abdominals gently hollowed to help control your center while you work the arms. If you have shoulder problems do not raise the arms above 90 degrees (follow the end of the sequence only). Beginners should master the moves without weights.

● To prepare, lengthen your spine, and take a deep breath in. Lengthen your arms and slowly raise them over your head. Make sure your elbows are bent and that your shoulders are relaxed and not lifted.

● Start to lower your arms down vertically and breathe out. Make sure your arms are slightly in front of your shoulders so your hands are still within your peripheral vision. Take a breath in.

inhale   exhale   inhale

● As you breathe out, bring the arms forward so the elbows meet in front of your body. Make sure the elbows don't drop as you perform this exercise.

● Press your arms back out again, keeping the elbows at right angles to your body. Keep your hands facing away from you. You should feel a stretch in the front of your chest.

● Start to straighten the arms out to the sides, remembering not to let your elbows drop and to keep your shoulders relaxed.

● As you complete the movement, turn your hands so they are facing down. Lengthen the neck, keep the ribs soft, and then relax.

| exhale | ▶ | inhale | ▶ | exhale | ▶ | breathe normally | ‖ |

walking and jogging

quads, hamstrings and core stability

Jogging is a gentle but effective means to aid circulation in the whole body. Performed with a Pilates focus, this exercise helps develop good alignment through ankles, knees, and hips. Think "tall" and hollow your lower abdominals, controlling your center as you move your limbs.

● Stand up straight and gently hollow your lower abdominals. Concentrate on keeping a neutral pelvis and lengthening the spine.

● Have your hands by your sides and lengthen your neck so your chin doesn't drop and you are not slouching. Keep your feet about hip width apart.

● Extend your right leg forward and begin to walk on the spot. Move your arms and relax your shoulders. Make sure you walk gently with a controlled movement.

inhale   ▶   exhale   ▶   inhale   ▶

● Try not to make a noise when walking, this will make sure the exercise is low impact. Start to walk on the balls of your feet.

● Increase the pace of your walking so it becomes a jog. Remember to keep your chin up, your neck lengthened, and your shoulders relaxed.

● Keep your chest well open as you jog gently on the spot. Bend your elbows and gently draw your shoulders back a little.

● As your upper back posture improves, you can challenge your shoulder girdle stability by making circles with your arms or raising them up and down.

exhale ▶ inhale exhale ‖ ▶ ‖

roll down against wall and sit

back extensors and core stability

This is a classic Pilates exercise, often used at the beginning or end of a class. It helps relieve muscle tension in your neck and shoulders, and improves the flexibility of your spine. Keep your hips over your knees as you roll—do not allow the pelvis to twist. Beginners should keep the knees bent throughout. You should not attempt this exercise if you have lower back problems.

● Start in the standing position with your feet apart and your knees relaxed. Breathe in and lengthen your spine. Pull in your abdominal muscles and gently lower your neck forward.

● Breathe out as you let your arms fall forward and your back curve. Relax your head and shoulders, and pay attention to your spine as it gently relaxes, curling over. Keep the movement gentle and controlled.

● Breathe in and start to roll slowly back up to the standing position. Imagine a string is attached to the crown of your head, pulling your body up in a straight line.

● Stand up straight and then stand tall on the tips of your feet. Imagine that you are leaning against a wall so your bottom doesn't push back or sway forward.

● Come back down so your feet are flat. Bend your knees and straighten them again. Then breathe in and contract your abdominals as you prepare to start rolling your head, neck, and back forward, as before.

● Bend your knees again, place your fingers on the floor for support, and kneel down. Put one leg back as you prepare to sit on the floor.

● Sit down in the cross-legged position and extend your arms at each side of your body. Lengthen your spine and neck, and relax.

exhale ▶ inhale exhale ‖ ▶ ‖

neck and shoulder stretch *mid and upper back extensors*

This exercise stretches the entire spine forward (into flexion). It is not suitable for those with neck and lower back problems, but can otherwise be used to release muscle tension. Try to keep your lower abdominals drawn in to support your spine and use your breathing to relax into the stretch.

● Begin the exercise cross-legged, with your spine upright and your arms out to the sides, fingertips pointing to the floor. Breathe in and lengthen the spine, keeping your lower abdominals contracted.

● Lean your head to the right and start to lift your right hand. Keep the left arm in position and the shoulders relaxed. Straighten the head again at this point.

● Continue to raise the hand, focusing on keeping the spine lengthened and the shoulders loose and soft.

● As the hand rises above horizontal, start to turn the palm in toward your head. At the same time, turn to face the hand as the arm hooks over.

| ■ | **inhale** | ▶ | **begin to exhale** | ▶ | | **exhale** | ▶ | **inhale** |

● Lightly hold the crown of your head. Take a breath here but do not pull on the neck, allowing the weight of the head to come forward for a gentle stretch.

● Breathe out as you bend from the neck. Let the spine gently roll down, using your hand for support. Continue the stretch as far as you can comfortably go. Breathe in and out again to deepen the stretch.

● When you have bent fully forward from the waist, take four breaths in the lowered position. Then, start to sit up again. Keep your hand on your head all the way up and don't release until you are upright.

● Return to the center position. Relax, lengthen the spine, and relax the shoulders. Now repeat the entire stretch on the other side.

exhale   ▶   ‖   inhale and exhale x 4   ▶   inhale   ▶   exhale

leg, spine, and hip stretch *back extensors and hip rotators*

This advanced sequence develops flexibility in the back and hips in preparation for advanced exercises. Do not attempt it if you have neck, hip, or lower back problems. Beginners should keep the knees bent. Do not use the open leg stretch unless you are an advanced exerciser.

● It is important to prepare properly for this exercise. Breathe in, lengthen the spine and loosen the shoulders. Relax your hips and sit into your pelvis. Beginners should sit on a cushion or low box.

● Keep you hands flat on the floor as you slide them forward. Move down from your neck, letting your spine curl gently and keeping your abdominals pulled into your spine.

● You will feel tension all along the spine as well as in the legs and buttocks. Continue the stretch as far as you can, but don't force yourself beyond your limits. Take six breaths at the farthest point of the stretch.

● Gently roll back up from your waist, stacking up the middle of the spine and finally the neck. Keep your lower abdominals contracted.

▶ **inhale** **exhale** ❚❚ **inhale and exhale x 6** ▶ **inhale** ▶

● Take a few seconds to make sure the spine is lengthened, the pelvis neutral, and the shoulders relaxed. Now, start to bring your legs out to the sides, keeping them straight. Beginners should not attempt this.

● Bring the arms forward over the legs and point the fingers in front of you at the floor.

● Start bending forward from the waist, letting your lower arms take your weight. Flatten the palms on the floor and keep them in place, bending at the elbows as the back lowers.

● Keep your abdominals drawn in. Do not force your hips or the forward bend of the spine. You should aim for a comfortable stretch.

exhale ▶ **inhale** **exhale** ▶ ▶ ▶

hip reach
spinal and hip rotators and adductors

This advanced exercise takes Pilates principles and applies them to a challenging stretch sequence. The focus of the stretch should be right at the fingertips with the rest of your arm and spine flowing behind. Aim for grace and flowing coordination. You should not attempt this exercise if you are a beginner or you suffer from lower back or hip problems.

● Stretch your legs out as far as possible and raise your arms up level with your shoulders, palms forward. Relax the shoulders, zip up, and make sure the pelvis is neutral. Start to twist to the left from the waist.

● As you twist, the arms should stay in line with each other. The whole of your upper body is pivoting from the waist, challenging hip muscles such as the obliques and the muscles of the lower back and upper leg.

● As you come over the left leg, twist your head to face behind you. Try to touch your toes. Use your breathing to enhance the stretch (lowering on the out breath). Keep the lower abdominals contracted.

● Now rise from the waist again. Bring your arms back in line with each other as your back straightens up. Keep your lower abdominals hollow as you stack up your spine.

■ ▶ inhale ▶ exhale ▶ inhale ▶ exhale ▶ inhale ▶

● Don't rest in the center position, move straight on to stretch on the other side. Twist from your waist to the right, keeping the arms in line with each other. Remember to keep focusing on your abdominals.

● As the head comes forward over the leg, turn it to face behind you. Reach your left hand to try to touch your toes. Extend the stretch as far as you can without forcing yourself beyond your natural range.

● Come back up to the center, untwisting and rising from the waist. Keep the arms outstretched and your fingers and toes pointed. Keep your lower abdominals drawn in to support your spine with each movement.

● Once back at the center, bring the legs together and the arms down to finish the exercise.

exhale   ▶   **inhale**   ▶   **exhale**   ▶

rainbow thoracic spine rotators and adductors

Focus on rooting your tailbone to the floor and hollowing your lower abdominals throughout this exercise. It is shown in advanced form here—do not strain at any point. Intermediate exercisers can perform a modified version, keeping the knees bent and closer together.

● Start with your legs straight and wide apart, as far as is comfortable. Point your toes away from you and extend your arms at your side. Breathe in and lengthen the spine.

● Start to turn your body to the left and then bend forward, keeping your abdominals drawn in to support your spine. Bend your right arm in front of you. Keep your shoulders relaxed.

● Rest the right elbow on the floor and turn your head to look along your left arm. Make sure the movement is from the waist and that the rest of your body stays still.

● Slowly start to twist back up again, bringing your left arm down and your right arm up. Keep your elbows soft and your lower abdominals working throughout the exercise.

■　　　　　　　　　II **begin to exhale**　　▶　　**exhale**　　▶　　**inhale**　　▶

● Now start to turn your body to the right. Keep your chin in neutral and don't lift it up.

● Lengthen the spine as you lean forward, and remember to keep the neck long as you turn to look at the raised hand.

● Contract your lower abdominals and start to lengthen your body back up again. Keep your toes pointed and your legs still. The movement should be in the waist.

● Come back up to the starting position with your arms stretched out to your sides and your head facing forward. Then take a deep breath in and out, and finally draw your legs and arms together.

exhale   ▶ inhale   exhale   ‖   ▶   ‖

hip flexor stretch rectus femoris, iliacus and adductors

As the name suggests, this routine focuses on stretching the muscles that cross the hip encouraging greater hip mobility. Beginners should hold the pose of the first image and not add the upper body twist. Keep the lower abdominals hollowed throughout and use padding for the knee as required. This exercise is not suitable if you have knee, hip, or lower back problems.

● Start with your right knee stretched out behind you and your left knee bent with your hands resting upon it. Breathe in and lengthen your spine.

● Lunge forward, keeping the head upright. Contract your abdominals so as not to compress your lower back. Reach your arms out and begin to turn to the left. Reach toward the floor only as far as is comfortable.

inhale   exhale   inhale

● Circle the right arm up over the head and stretch your right leg straight, keeping it close to the floor. Place the palm of your left hand on the floor and turn your head to face toward it.

● Now, start to sit back onto your right leg as you bring your arm back over your head again. Keep your shoulders down as you move your arm and think "tall" into your spine keeping your abdominals drawn in.

● As you sit back on your right leg, your left leg should form a 90 degree angle to the floor. Bring your right arm back down to your right side.

● Looking forward again, bring both hands to rest on your left knee. Repeat this exercise, beginning with the left knee stretched out behind you.

exhale   inhale   ▶   exhale   inhale   II   ▶   II

inside and outside hip stretch

hip rotators and back extensors

This stretch targets the deep rotators of the hip. It also gives the whole spine from the base of the neck to the tailbone (coccyx) a gentle yet effective stretch. The version shown is intermediate. Beginners should bend the top leg only (keep the other straight underneath it) and only bring the spine forward a little, omitting the leg scissoring.

● Sit upright with your back straight and your fingertips resting on the floor. Bend both your knees and then cross your left leg over your right leg so it is resting on your right thigh. Keep your toes pointed.

● Drawing your abdominals into your spine, start to curve your neck and waist forward, moving your hands forward as you bend over. Bend over as far as is comfortable, resting your chin on your knee if possible.

● In this forward position, take six breaths and expand as much of the body as possible. Breathe out and release any tension starting from the head, then the neck, and finally the shoulders.

● Now, begin to curve your torso back up again so you reach a sitting position. Keep your back straight as you place your hands behind you and begin to lean back.

| ■ inhale | ‖ exhale | ▶ inhale and exhale x 6 | exhale | ▶ |

● Uncross your legs, extend them, and then push them apart as far as possible. Keep your toes pointed. Hold this pose and then open them as far as you comfortably can. Hold this pose briefly as you breathe in and out.

● Begin to close your legs again, bend your knees, and this time cross your right leg over your left thigh. Use your arms to support you and keep your neck relaxed.

● Start to come forward with your body again and bring the arms forward, too. Be careful not to force or push your body in any way, and only bend forward as much as is comfortable for you.

● Hold this position for up to six breaths, relaxing on the out breath and expanding on the in breath. Draw in your abdominals as you sit up slowly and relax.

inhale and exhale   ▶ **inhale**   **exhale**   ‖ **inhale and exhale**

curl, twist, and airplane

This exercise is a demanding workout for the whole abdominal group (especially the external and internal obliques). Beginners should build strength by practising the simple rolling back action at the start of the sequence, progressing through arms bent to the full version shown at the end. Do not attempt this exercise if you have lower back problems.

● Sit upright with your knees bent and your feet flat on the floor. If this is uncomfortable, sit on a cushion. Have your arms rounded in front of you and above your knees. Breathe in and contract your lower abdominals.

● Breathe out and gradually roll back, lowering your back only as far as you can maintain good abdominal control.

● Turn your body to the left in mid "sit back." Release the tension between your shoulders and engage the stomach muscles to keep your back supported. Move your arms and head together as you turn to the left.

● Then come back to the center and twist to the right. Use your lower abdominals to keep the pose smooth. Return to the center and repeat this movement on both sides three times.

■ **inhale**　　　　Ⅱ **exhale**　　　▶ **exhale**　　　▶ **inhale**　　　**exhale**

● After these repetitions, return to the center. Keep leaning back and begin to open your arms out to the sides. Twist to the left, putting the left hand down on the floor and the right hand parallel pointing up.

● Keep the arms straight and stretched and come back to the horizontal position. Remember to keep your shoulders soft and relaxed all the time.

● Now, twist to the right, turning your head toward your right hand and raising your left arm into the air as you turn. Keep your buttocks firmly on the floor and concentrate on making this a controlled, slow movement.

● Reach your right hand down to the floor and feel the work in your oblique muscles. Repeat this airplane exercise on both sides.

exhale ▶ **inhale** **exhale** ❙❙ ▶ ❙❙

outstretched wings and roll down *and hip flexors*

The outstretched wings works your waist (internal and external oblique externals) and performed with control, helps you develop core stability. Beginners should master the curl, twist, and airplane before moving on to this exercise. Do not attempt this exercise if you have lower back problems.

● Begin this exercise in the airplane position with your arms extended and the right fingers on the floor. Have your knees bent, your feet flat on the floor, and your lower abdominals engaged to support your back.

● Breathe in and float arms up above your head. Keep leaning to the right and keep your head pointing to the right, too.

● Raise your left leg as you move your arms down again. Breathe out and pull in your lower abdominals as you extend this leg. Keep the lower back curved and only extend your leg as far as it feels comfortable.

● Repeat this exercise with the right leg. Remember to keep the supporting leg bent and to keep your buttocks on the floor. Turn your body to the left and raise your right arm in the air. Repeat up to four times on each side.

⏸ inhale ▶ exhale ▶ inhale ⏸

● Now, as you breath out, contract your lower abdominals and raise both legs in the air with the knees bent and the toes pointed. Keep your arms rounded and above your head, and your abdominal muscles pulled in.

● As you begin to roll back, straighten your legs out in front of you. Slowly roll back, vertebra by vertebra. Keep your legs raised off the floor at quite a high angle. You can have them at a lower angle as you build your strength.

● Lower your torso onto the floor as you begin to bend your knees. Lower your arms by your sides. Make sure you do not arch the spine; this will strain your back. Keep your neck relaxed.

● Finish this exercise with your back flat on the floor, your knees at a right angle, and your arms extended by your sides. Repeat this rolling-down exercise four times. Then put both feet back on the floor and relax.

begin to exhale　　　▶　**exhale**　　　**exhale**　　　ǁ　　▶　　ǁ

upper ab curl *abdominal muscles*

This exercise works all four muscles of the abdominal group (rectus abdominis, internal and external obliques, and transversus). The transversus abdominis, responsible for abdominal hollowing, should be gently drawn in toward your spine before you begin to curl. This is what turns a generic sit-up into a powerful Pilates move. Try to keep your pelvis steady and your lower back neutral.

● Start this exercise lying on the floor with your knees bent. Have your arms behind your head to support your neck. Breathe in and lengthen the spine.

● Lift the head and shoulders off the floor. Curl up one vertebra at a time to a comfortable position. Scoop your stomach muscles in to support your lower back and keep your pelvis in the neutral position.

● Bring your right hand forward toward your hip. Keep the other arm behind your head to make sure your head is in the correct position. Lengthen and relax your neck. Fix your gaze slightly above your knees.

● Extend your right arm so it is level with your hip. Then start to bring the other arm down, making sure you keep your neck in the same position. Beginners can support the head throughout swopping hands.

‖ exhale ▶ inhale ▶ exhale ▶

● As you extend your left arm down toward your hip, start to bring the right arm up toward your head again.

● After you have stretched your left arm forward, start to bring it back toward your neck again. Keep your spine in neutral and your lower abdominals drawn in.

● Then put both hands behind your neck and roll back down on the floor to relax.

● This exercise can be repeated as many times as you like, but you must be careful not to strain your neck and shoulders as you perform it.

inhale   ▶ begin to exhale   exhale   ‖   ▶   ‖

intermediate

starlight abdominal muscles

This exercise gives all four of the abdominal muscle groups an intense workout. However, it needs to be performed carefully. Avoid straining the neck and shoulders when curling up and make sure the lower back does not arch away from the floor at any time. If you have any neck or lower back problems do not attempt this exercise.

● Begin this exercise lying down with your knees bent and your feet flat on the floor. Have your hands clasped behind your head with your elbows slightly raised. Breathe in and lengthen the spine.

● Breathe out and engage the lower abdominal muscles before you begin to curl up. Gradually, raise the head, neck, and shoulders from the floor and support your head with your hands.

● Lift your right knee up so the leg is at a 90 degree angle to your body. Keep your head up high, your neck relaxed, and your shoulders down.

● Contract your lower abdominals as you raise the left leg up so it is parallel with your right leg. Keep your toes pointing out. Concentrate on keeping your jaw relaxed and your chin dropped.

■   ‖ **exhale**   ▶   **inhale**   ▶   **exhale**   ▶

● Begin to curl up as you bring your knees toward your chin. Keep the movement controlled and your back pressed into the floor. Curl up into as small a shape as is comfortable while contracting your lower abdominals.

● Breathe out and start to uncurl. Roll your upper back down onto the floor as far as the bottom of your shoulders and move your knees away from you.

● Bring your legs to the ground with your toes touching the floor. Don't lower your legs this far if you can feel your back straining. Only lower your legs as far as you can without arching your back.

● Pull your lower abdominals in tightly and keep your head up as high as possible. Repeat this sequence four times and finish curled up ready for the next exercise.

inhale ▶ **begin to exhale** **exhale** ❚❚ ▶ ❚❚

crisscross
oblique abdominals and hip flexors

This original Pilates exercise is excellent for strengthening the abdominals and training upper and lower body coordination. Beginners can start by rotating the upper body only and keeping both feet on the floor. Progress to holding the feet in the air and then gradually begin to straighten them as your strength improves. Do not attempt this exercise if you have neck and lower back problems.

● Lie on your back with your hands behind your head. Contract your lower abdominals then lift your head and bend your knees into your chest. Keep your elbows extended as much as possible.

● Start to extend you right leg out; as you do so, begin to twist your upper body so your right elbow is aiming for your left knee. Keep hollowing the lower abdominals and allow the lower back to flatten slightly.

● Make sure you are lifting from below your shoulder in order to reach the knee and not twisting from the shoulder socket. Bring the elbow so it almost touches the left knee. Hold the position and breathe out.

● As you start to move the right leg back, begin to extend the opposite leg out in front of you.

II inhale   ▶   exhale   ▶   inhale   ▶

● Aim your left elbow for your right knee, but imagine that your center is anchored to the floor so you don't rock your body from hip to hip.

● As you extend your left leg, do not allow it to drop too low in front of you. You can maintain control of the leg position by squeezing your buttocks and doing the exercise slowly.

● Concentrate on lifting and twisting from your waist. You should feel the work above and below your waistline.

● When the left leg is fully extended, hold the stretch and exhale completely. Complete up to 10 times, then pull your knees into your chest to relax back on the floor.

exhale ▶ exhale inhale ▶ exhale ❚❚

waist twists *quadratus lumborum*

This exercise works the oblique abdominals and stretches a major side flexor of the spine and the spinal rotators. It also increases the mobility of the spine especially in the thoracic area. Beginners or those who have had back problems should keep their feet on the floor and only attempt the version shown in the first four images. Do not attempt this exercise if you have current back problems.

● Start the exercise by lying on your back with your feet flat on the floor and your knees bent. Breathe in deeply and lengthen the spine.

● Stretch your arms out to the side so they are parallel with your shoulders. Pause.

● As you breathe out, drop your knees comfortably to your left side while turning your head in the other direction. Use your breathing to increase the stretch and keep your lower abdominals contracted.

● Return your legs to the center and then repeat the exercise on the other side, dropping your knees to the right and turning your head to the left.

| inhale | ‖ | ▶ | exhale | ▶ | inhale | ▶ |

● For an advanced level of Pilates, begin this exercise with your knees in the air at right angles to your body. Place a tennis ball between your knees and grip it.

● Then twist to the left with your legs, keeping the ball in the same position, and turn your head to the right.

● Return your legs to the starting position and then repeat on the other side. Concentrate on lengthening the spine and neck as you do this exercise, and make sure you twist from the waist and not the shoulders.

● Inhaling, refill your lungs, feel your chest expand as you return to the center and relax.

inhale   ▶   exhale   ▶   inhale   exhale ▶   inhale   ‖

creating energy

hip lift

oblique abdominals and glutes

The principal challenge here is to keep your body balanced and steady while the leg is elevated.
You will feel your pelvis tip to the side or sway as each leg comes up. Try to keep your pelvis and
spine aligned by using your hands at your side. Beginners should practice just raising the heel
before progressing to straightening the leg. Do not attempt this exercise if you have back problems.

● Begin the exercise in the relaxation position, with the feet flat on the floor and the knees bent. Beginners should aim to lift the heel only at first, before progressing to lifting the leg.

● On an out breath, pull in the lower abdominals and start to lift the pelvis up to wherever is comfortable. Now start to lift the left foot off the ground.

● Continue reaching up with the left leg until it is pointing about 40 degrees from the floor. Pause here for a second and breathe in.

● As you breathe out, contract your lower abdominals and lower the left leg to the floor again. When it reaches the floor, pause again and breathe in.

■   inhale   ▶   exhale   inhale   ‖   exhale   ▶   inhale

● Now repeat the sequence with the right leg. Remember to lift the leg on an outbreath and pause when you reach the straight leg position.

● Breathe in as you hold the position. Feel the leg lengthening at the knee, pulling away from the hips, which remain steady and square.

● Breathe out as you lower the right leg to the floor. Do this with control; don't just let it collapse.

● With both feet grounded, bring the pelvis back to the floor. As with the feet, don't let the pelvis collapse. Lower it slowly and gently, keeping the lower abdominals hollowed.

exhale　　　　▶　　　　inhale　　▐▐　　exhale　　　　　　▶　　　　　　breathe normally

advanced pelvic lifts
gluts, oblique abdominals

This exercise further challenges your core stability. You'll need to work hard to maintain rib and pelvic alignment as you lower and lift your leg. Make sure you keep the weight on your shoulders rather than the neck, and avoid over arching the back. This routine is good for strengthening the buttock muscles (gluteals) and also works the hip rotators. Do not attempt this exercise if you have lower back problems.

● Lie on your back with your hands parallel to your body. Have your feet flat, knees bent, and your heels together. Breathe in and lengthen the spine and neck.

● Raise the pelvis, keeping the shoulders on the floor. Lift your bottom off the floor so it is in line with your legs. Make sure that you keep the ribs soft and relaxed.

● Then extend and lift the right leg, keeping your back straight and your hips raised. Flex the foot and support your body through your arms. Keep the lower abs contracted. Stop if your lower back hurts at any point.

● Raise your right leg up farther so it is in line with your hips. Keep the foot flexed and your spine straight.

■   ‖ **exhale**   ▶ **inhale**   **exhale** ▶ **inhale**   ▶

● If you want to continue to a more advanced level, bring your leg right up so it is at a right angle with your body. Keep the supporting leg bent with the foot flat on the floor.

● Start to lower your leg gradually down again, pointing it as you do so. Keep your bottom raised off the ground and don't arch your back. Keep your lower abdominals contracted and your pelvis steady.

● Bring the leg all the way down to the floor and then start to lower your body back down again.

● Keep your pelvis lifted as you lower your buttocks down last. Put your heels together and relax. Repeat this sequence with your left leg. Work through your spine and lower the pelvis and buttocks last.

exhale   inhale   ▶   exhale   inhale   ❚❚   ▶   ❚❚

tree climb

hamstrings and gastrocnemius

This is an advanced hamstring and calf stretch performed in lying and sitting positions. It requires good abdominal control to keep the pelvis steady. Beginners may attempt a modified version by keeping the knees bent in both parts of the exercise. Always contract the lower abdominals to support the back. Do not attempt this exercise if you have lower back problems.

● Begin the sequence lying flat on the floor with your arms by your sides and your palms facing down. Inhale and lengthen the spine.

● Contract your lower abdominals as you lift your right knee. Lift both arms toward your raised knee. Bring your knee back to 90 degrees to the body, and place your hands on the front of the knee, flexing your foot to point.

● Pull the knee back into the chest and take the hands onto the inside of the thigh, just below the knee. Keep drawing in your lower abdominals as you straighten your raised leg to a comfortable vertical position.

● Carefully straighten the extended leg, bringing it in toward your body. Flex the heel so you feel a stretch—not a strain—in the hamstrings and calf muscles. You should not feel anything in the back.

| ■ | inhale | exhale | ▶ | inhale | ▶ | breathe normally | ‖ |

● Now lift your head and shoulders from the floor toward your raised leg. As you do so, slowly move your hands up your leg to avoid straining your neck and shoulders. Keep your lower abdominals pulled in to your spine and make sure your pelvis is level.

● Continue raising your body and moving your hands up your leg until they are gripping the calf muscles just below the ankle. Both legs should be straight with toes pointed. Inhale deeply and hold the pose. Keep the abdominals engaged and pelvis square.

● Now release the stretch and walk your hands back down the leg as you slowly lower your back toward the floor. Once your hands are on the back of your thigh again, bend your leg and bring the foot down to rest flat on the floor.

● Extend your leg once it is back on the floor, making sure both toes point away from the body. Bring your arms down to your sides with palms facing the floor. Relax and breathe deeply, then repeat the exercise with the other leg.

exhale   **inhale**   ‖   **exhale**   **inhale**   ▶   **breathe normally**   ‖

adductor stretch *and hip rotators*

This exercise stretches the inner thigh. To maintain good pelvic alignment, you will need to coordinate the deep hip and abdominal muscles. Aim for a gentle stretch in the inner thighs—do not push or force the legs, and don't arch the back. Beginners should perform the stretch by keeping both feet on the floor, allowing the knees to drop out while keeping the pelvis steady. At intermediate level, the knees should be kept bent throughout. The straight leg version shown is highly advanced. Do not attempt this exercise if you have lower back, hip, or knee problems.

● Lie on your back with your knees bent and your feet flat on the floor. Take a deep breath in and lengthen the spine.

● Lift your right leg up so it is at a 90 degree angle to your body. Then bring your left leg up so it is parallel to it. Keep your abdominals drawn in and your pelvis steady.

● Grip your knees with your hands and start to open your legs as far apart as you can. Activate the abs to avoid arching your back off the floor as you do this. Keep your neck lengthened and relaxed.

● Change the grip to the inside of your thighs and extend your legs out straight as far as you find comfortable. There should be no pain in your knees. Point your toes out. Hold this position for a few breaths.

■   ‖ inhale   ▶   begin to exhale   ▶   exhale   ▶

● Then close your legs, keeping them straight so they are at a 90 degree angle to your body. Keep your toes pointed and your back firmly on the floor. Breathe in.

● Lower your legs back down again, keeping your abdominals pulled in to your spine as you do. Remember, this is a highly advanced stretch, you should not push into discomfort.

● Bend your knees from this position and grip the outside of your knees to pull them up to the center again. Then put both of your arms on the floor, parallel to your body with your palms facing down.

● Lower the right leg to the floor and then the left leg. Take a deep breath in and then out. Relax.

inhale ▶ exhale inhale ❚❚ ▶ ❚❚

jackknife with back stretch
abdominals and hip flexors

This advanced exercise is shown below in its ideal form. When you first try the rollover, don't straighten your legs or force them back farther than is comfortable. The roll hyperflexes the upper spine and neck so keep your lower abdominals hollow throughout the sequence. Don't attempt this exercise if you have neck or lower back problems, or have had a spinal disc injury.

● Start the exercise in the relaxation position, with the feet flat on the floor and the knees bent. Spend a few seconds focusing on your spine and contract your lower abdominals to prepare support for your back.

● Bring first the left leg and then the right up from the hip, until the knee forms a 90 degree angle. Keep your lower abdominals engaged and your pelvis steady.

● Now straighten the lower leg with the upper leg. Pause here and breathe in before continuing with the roll.

● Let your legs come over your body as you exhale. Maintain control by bringing your spine off the floor vertebrae by vertebrae. Rest on your upper back, not your neck. Straighten your leg only if it is comfortable.

■ inhale   ▶ exhale   ‖ inhale   exhale   ▶   inhale   ▶

● Continue backward until your toes touch the floor. Then bring your knees toward your shoulders. Pause and breathe in here.

● As you breathe out, extend the legs again. Use your hands by your side to keep you steady, but focus your energy and concentration on your hips and abdominals.

● Bring your feet up, keeping the legs straight until you reach the upright position. Reverse the beginning of the exercise now, bending at the knees to come to a 90 degree angle.

● To finish the rollover, lower one and then the other foot onto the floor. Focus on keeping your lower abdominals drawn in and your spine lengthened.

exhale   ▶   ‖   inhale   exhale

leg switch

abdominals and hip flexors

Although the focus of movement in this exercise is the legs, the hard work takes place in the abdominal muscles, which need to be activated to support the spine. Gently press your spine into the floor without tucking your pelvis under. Don't arch the lower back and avoid this exercise if you have neck or lower back problems.

● Start in the relaxation position, with the feet flat and the knees bent. Place your hands behind your head. Breathe in as you prepare, and contract your lower abdominals to gently flatten the spine into the floor.

● Breathe out as you lift one and then the other leg up so the lower leg is horizontal. Now take your legs up to the vertical.

● Breathe in at the vertical position, then breathe out as you lift your head and shoulders up off the floor. Keep your abdominals engaged and your pelvis steady.

● Keeping your head raised, lower your left leg. Keep your spine straight and don't let your back arch or your shoulder blades come off the floor. Lower your leg only as far as you can keep your abdominals pulling in.

■ inhale   ▶ exhale   ‖ inhale   exhale   ▶ inhale   exhale

● Bring the left leg back to join the right leg. Now allow the right leg to lower to the floor. Do not allow your pelvis to roll or twist.

● Keep the toes pointed out as your right leg reaches horizontal. The leg shouldn't actually touch the floor at the horizontal level.

● Now bring the right leg back up to the vertical and bend at the knees to bring both legs to a 90 degree angle.

● Continue to breathe out as you lower your feet to the floor and relax the pelvis and the spine.

inhale   exhale   ▶   inhale   exhale   ‖   inhale   ▶   exhale

arm reaches and arcs

pectoralis major

This exercise works in two ways: the shoulder stretches relieve tension in the upper back while the
arc movements open the front of the chest, stretching and strengthening the pectoral muscles,
biceps, and anterior deltoids. Using weights will add resistance to help build strength. Do not
attempt this exercise if you have shoulder problems.

● Start on your back with your knees
bent, shoulders relaxed, and your
pelvis neutral. Have your arms straight
by your side. You can add arm weights
if you are at an intermediate or
advanced stage. Breathe in.

● Tuck your chin in without lifting
your head so the back of your neck is
lengthened. Begin to lift both your
arms straight up in the air so they are
at a 90 degree angle to your body.

● Now, lift your right shoulder so
your right arm reaches beyond your
left one. Keep your palms facing in.
Hold, and then slowly melt the
shoulder back into the floor. Repeat
using the left shoulder.

● Bend your arms at the elbows and
concentrate on opening your chest
and shoulders as you form a circle
with your arms. Touch your fingers
together and imagine that you are
hugging a big tree.

■　　　　　　　　　II exhale　　　　　▶　　　inhale　　　　　▶　　begin to inhale　　　　▶

● Then open your arms out to the sides so they are parallel with your shoulders. Keep your arms bent and don't touch the floor with them.

● Start to raise your arms back up together again. Remember to keep your spine lengthened throughout this exercise, and be careful not to hyper-extend your elbows or lose your lengthened neck curve.

● Complete the circle by touching your fingertips together again. Make sure the movement is controlled with your neck relaxed. Do not flare your ribs at any stage during this routine or allow your hips or knees to move.

● Finish the routine by gently lowering your arms back down to the floor again. Remove your arm weights and relax.

inhale   ▶ exhale   inhale   ‖   ▶   ‖

arm switch and triceps curls and triceps

This exercise challenges the stability of the ribcage and shoulder girdle. Focus on keeping your spine aligned on the floor. Don't let your back arch or your ribs flare as your arms go over your head. If you feel any strain, make the movements smaller. Do not perform this exercise if you have shoulder problems. For the tricep curl, focus on the elbow joint, keeping the upper arm still.

● Begin in the relaxation position with your arms vertical. Keep your elbows soft—don't lock them. Breathe in as you prepare to move your arms.

● Breathe out as you lower both arms straight down in parallel with your body. The left arm goes back behind your head, the right comes down beside your waist. Keep the wrists in line with the rest of the arms.

● Breathe in as you aim to take the arm to the horizontal, without letting it touch the floor. Breathe out and contract your abdominals as you start to raise your arms back to the vertical.

● As your arms come together, take a breath, and concentrate on correcting your posture—lengthen the spine, loosen the elbows, and soften the shoulders. Now breathe out as you begin to lower your arms again.

■ ▶ **inhale**   **exhale**   ‖ **inhale** ▶ **exhale**   ‖ **inhale** ▶ **exhale**

● This time, lower each arm in the opposite direction. Again, try to keep the wrists straight, don't flare your ribs, and keep your spine lengthened.

● Breathe out as you lower your arms, breathe in when they reach the horizontal position, and then breathe out as you raise them back to vertical. Repeat this exercise eight times.

● Now place your right hand behind your left elbow to support it for the tricep curl. The tricep is the muscle on the back of the upper arm. Slowly lift the weight back up to the vertical, pivoting around the elbow.

● Take the weight down to ear level and then raise it back up to vertical. Now repeat with the other arm. Do up to eight sets of this exercise.

ǁ inhale   ▶ exhale   ǁ inhale   ▶   exhale   inhale

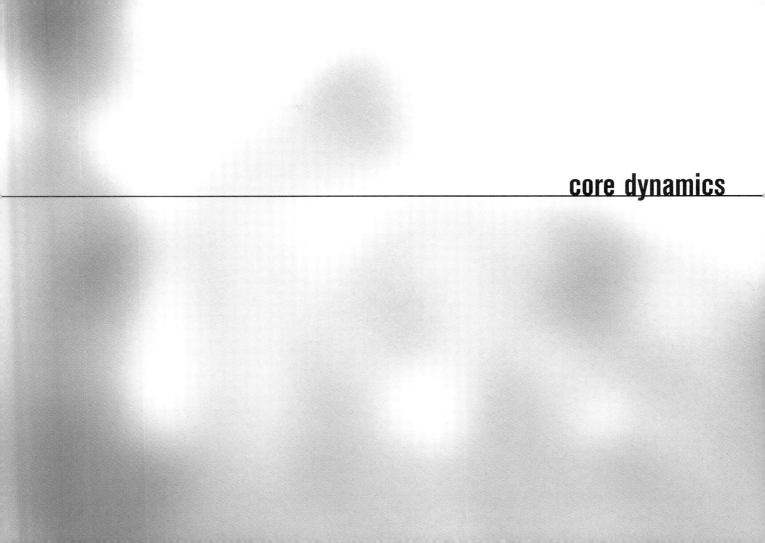

core dynamics

intermediate
abductor lift

This exercise works the buttock muscles (gluteals), while the muscles along the back of your legs (hamstrings and gastrocnemius) are lengthening. It also challenges your core control in the shoulder girdle and pelvis as you work to keep your torso steady. Intermediate and advanced exercisers can use leg weights to add resistance. Beginners can attempt a less demanding version, keeping the working leg bent and the lift small. Do not attempt this if you have knee or lower back problems.

- Start on your left side, with your knees bent at a right angle to your body and your right hand on your hip. Have your head resting on a towel or small pillow, as this will help to keep your neck straight.

- Breathe in and begin to lift your right leg up. Breathe out and stretch your leg straight in line with your body. Keep your lower abs contracted.

- Now flex the right foot and point the toes to the floor. Raise your leg a few inches and then lower it again. Repeat this up to four times, depending on strength and stamina.

- Pull your leg forward in front of you to hip level. Raise your leg up an inch from this position and then lower it.

II inhale   exhale   inhale   ▶   exhale   ▶

● Take your right leg back to join the left leg. Be careful not to arch your back at all. Keep your abdominals engaged, your spine lengthened, and your eyes straight ahead.

● Now slide your right leg over the left leg, and flex and point the foot. Repeat up to four times.

● Keep your right hand on your right hip and remember to keep your abdominals contracted so that your spine is supported. Then begin to stretch both legs out so they are aligned with the rest of your body.

● Bring your right hand in front of your stomach with the palm down. Keep your heels together and rise onto your left elbow. Turn over and repeat this exercise on the other side.

inhale   ▶   exhale   inhale   ‖   ▶   ‖

frog *hips and knees*

This exercise engages your upper back muscles (latissimus dorsi, serratus anterior, and posterior) It also challenges you to stabilize your ribcage and work your inner and outer thigh muscles and hip rotators. Focus on supporting your lower back with your abdominals and keep your pelvis stable. Do not attempt this exercise if you have shoulder, lower back, or knee problems.

● You can begin this exercise in the final position described in the glass table. Your body should be in a straight line, with your torso raised on your left elbow and your right hand in front for support.

● Breathe in and bring your knees and heels up so that you make a frog leg shape with them. Keep your lower abdominals contracted so that your pelvis remains steady and your back does not arch.

● As you breathe out, extend the right leg up straight, with your foot flexed. Keep your lower ribs lifted off the floor and your neck relaxed. Only lift as far as feels comfortable and you can keep your pelvis still.

● Bring your heels back together again. Remember to keep your chest open and your shoulders down away from the ears.

■   ‖ inhale   ▶ exhale   ▶ inhale   ▶

● Breathe out and extend both legs out so that your body is in a straight line. Lengthen from the top of the head and then bring your right leg forward and your underneath leg back, toes pointed, engaging your lower abs.

● Then bring the underneath (left) leg forward and the top (right) leg back. As you do this scissor movement, do not roll your body back and forth. Your hips should be steady and only the legs should move.

● Only stretch your legs back and forth as far as is comfortable and do not strain them. Keep a long neck and make sure your spine is lengthened and shoulders relaxed.

● Breathe in and join your legs together again. Engage your stomach muscles and then raise your legs together slightly and put them back down on the floor again. Repeat the whole routine on your right side.

exhale   inhale   ▶ exhale   exhale   ❚❚   ▶   ❚❚

diamond press

This shoulder press will stretch the front of the spine and thighs as you kick. Beginners should study the first two images and attempt the leg kick with the forearms and lower ribs on the floor. Do not attempt this exercise if you have lower back or knee problems.

● Begin this sequence lying on your stomach, with your forehead resting on your hands and your legs outstretched, toes pointing away from the body. With your elbows extended to your sides, your arms should form a diamond shape.

● Lift your lower abs up toward your spine and push up from the palms of your hands. Continue the raise until your arms are straight and your head is facing upright. Repeat this raise three or four times. You will feel a stretch along the abdomen.

● Holding yourself up on your arms with your head facing forward, slowly raise your right foot, flexing at the knee. Keep your foot pointed toward the ceiling to form a 90 degree angle if this is comfortable.

● Now lower the leg and repeat the exercise with the other leg, remembering to keep your foot pointed throughout the movement. Repeat the raise on both legs three or four times.

■   **inhale**   **exhale**   II   **inhale**   **exhale**   ▶   **inhale**   II   **exhale**

● Lower both legs back down to rest on the floor, keeping your body raised on your extended arms. Now bring both legs up together to point your toes to the ceiling. Do not bring the legs back more than feels comfortable. Keep the lower abs contracted.

● Lengthen your neck and look up a little toward the ceiling. Do not continue with this move if you feel any discomfort, especially in your lower back, knees, or neck.

● Release the stretch. Lower your head forward toward the ground, at the same time extending your legs to rest your feet on the floor.

● Bring your elbows to rest flat on the floor in the diamond position. Bring your head down to rest on the backs of your hands. Relax and breathe deeply, expand your ribs and let the spine lengthen and relax.

inhale   exhale   ‖   inhale   exhale   ▶   breathe deeply   ‖

salute, reach, and swim

A perfect workout for the back, this original Pilates exercise strengthens all the muscles along your spine and increases the mobility of your upper back (thoracic spine) and shoulder girdle. Although the lower back is extended, keep your lower abdominals contracted throughout. Think "long in the limbs" and "lifted through the center." Do not use this exercise if you have shoulder or lower back problems.

- ● Lie on your stomach with your forehead touching the floor and your chin tucked in. Have your arms by your side with your hands resting palms up. Lengthen your spine and pull in your abdominal muscles.

- ● Begin to turn your palms into your body and start to lift your head slowly. Make sure you use your abdominal muscles to lift your navel off the floor and squeeze your buttocks together a little to help keep your pelvis steady.

- ● Turn your palms to face the floor, keep your head up, and bring both arms up at a right angle to your head in a saluting gesture. Make sure you don't let your elbows drop. Repeat this exercise four times.

- ● After the fourth repetition, bring your arms back to the side of your body. Now bring the arms up in a straight line in front of you and hold the stretch. Repeat this exercise four times too.

■   **inhale** ▶   **exhale**   **inhale** ▶   **exhale**   ▶

● After you've finished this sequence, place your forehead on the floor again. Inhale, pulling your navel into your spine as you start to bring your right arm and your left arm up into the air simultaneously.

● If possible, lift both legs off the floor when doing this exercise. Do not lift too high—the lengthening of the limbs is more important. Lower the limbs to change to the other side. Work from your hips, not your knees.

● Keep the movement slow and controlled, making sure your arms and legs are as straight as possible. Do not allow your stomach to drop as this will put strain on your lower back. Keep your lower abs contracted.

● When you have finished, bend your elbows and put your forehead onto your arms. Keep your neck lengthened, and relax.

inhale ▶ **exhale** **inhale** ▶ **exhale** ▶ II

hamstring curls and double leg kicks

This original Pilates exercise works the buttocks (gluteals) and hamstrings, and stretches the front of the thigh (quadriceps). Aim to contract your glutes before the kick. This helps you work from the hip, not the knee. Keep you lower abdominals contracted so that your back does not overarch and your pelvis does not twist. Avoid this exercise if you have knee or lower back problems.

● Begin with your forehead on your fingers and your body outstretched. Take a deep breath in, contract your lower abs and lengthen the spine.

● Keeping your head in the same position, lengthen your left leg and breathe out as you begin to lift it about an inch from the floor.

● Take a breath in as you begin to bend the right knee up toward your bottom. Make sure that the opposite leg remains on the floor. Keep your stomach contracted, your shoulders relaxed and your neck lengthened.

● Bring the leg up so that it is at a right angle to your body, if this is comfortable, and then as you breathe out flex the foot. Breathe in, point your foot, and then bring the leg back down again. Repeat with the other leg.

| inhale | ▶ | exhale | ▶ | inhale | ▶ | exhale | inhale ▶ |

● Begin on the right leg again, contract your lower abs, bend your knee, and bring the leg up hard to your right buttock. Take it back to a right angle, flex the foot, and then bring it back again.

● On an outbreath, lower your leg down again with your foot pointing out. Keep your upper thighs and knees glued together as you kick to engage the hamstring and buttock muscles, and help your core control.

● Repeat using the other leg. Keep your abdominal muscles contracted throughout this exercise and lengthen your body from the crown of your head so that you maintain a long neck to support the weight of your head.

● When you have finished this sequence, sit back on your heels to release your lower back. Then push back into the half cat.

exhale   inhale ▶   exhale   ▶   inhale ▶   exhale   ▶ ❚❚   ▶   ❚❚

leg circles and beats
gluteus maximus and hip rotators

This exercise works the gluteals, hamstrings, and hip rotators. It challenges your core control as you have to keep your lower abdominals contracted to stop your lower back and shoulders overworking. Beginners should study the first two images and keep the leg raise and circle small. Progress to the more advanced versions shown as your strength and stamina improve. Do not attempt this exercise if you have lower back problems made worse by arching your lower spine.

● Begin the sequence lying on your stomach with your head resting on your hands. Keep your shoulders relaxed and breathe in.

● Concentrate on your breath out as you lengthen the right leg and then begin to lift it up. Keeping the leg straight, start to circle it as if you were drawing small circles on the wall behind you. Do up to eight reps.

● Increase the size of each circle as you progress. Repeat with the other leg. If the back is strong enough circle both legs at the same time, but keep the legs low, and stop if you feel any discomfort in your lower back.

● For the "beats," slowly lift both legs together and open and close them in a scissor-like action. Flex and point the feet as you open and close your legs, making sure you keep your lower abs and glutes strongly contracted.

inhale	exhale	inhale and exhale x 4	inhale	exhale

● Repeat this exercise up to eight times, first with pointed feet, then with flexed feet, and finally crossing your feet over each other.

● Keep your feet together and bend your knees out. Breathe out, contract your lower abs, and raise your knees about an inch above the floor. Keep your pubic bone on the floor and do not allow your back to overarch.

● Lift your legs so that they are at a 90 degree angle to your body. Then lift the legs from the hips and down again. Make sure that your lower abdominals are supporting your back throughout. Stop if you feel any discomfort.

● Lower your legs to a 45 degree angle and raise from the hips again. Keep your heels together and repeat this exercise eight times. Relax.

inhale   exhale   ▶   ❚❚   exhale   ▶   inhale   exhale   ■

quad and hamstring stretch *hamstrings*

This exercise stretches the front and back of your thighs (quads and hamstrings). It is important to keep your abdominals pulled in and concentrate on keeping your back aligned in its natural curves (in neutral). Do not attempt this exercise if you have knee problems. If you have lower back problems or are a beginner, only attempt the first part of the stretch for the front of the thigh.

● Lie on your right side with your legs bent at a 90 degree angle. Rest your head on your right arm. You can place a pillow underneath for extra comfort. Place your left arm on your hip. Breathe in and lengthen the spine.

● Slowly lift the left leg off the floor and then begin to move it back toward your buttocks.

● Clasp your ankle with your left hand and pull your left leg back so that it is touching, or near, your buttocks. Keep your shoulders relaxed and the other knee firmly on the floor.

● Place your left hand on your left thigh and move your leg around to the front of your body.

| ■ | II inhale | ▶ exhale | ▶ inhale | ▶ |

● Start to straighten the left leg out in front of you, moving your hand up for support. Pull the straight leg up as far as possible. Contract your lower abs and only pull the leg as far as you can feel a comfortable stretch.

● Now move your left leg back toward your right leg, bending the knee as you do so. Keep your chest open and your shoulders relaxed as you perform this exercise.

● Bend the leg back toward your buttocks, as before. Grip your ankle with your left hand and feel the stretch all along your thigh. Keep your lower abs pulled in and do not allow your spine to overarch.

● Allow your left leg to rest on your right leg again. Pause and repeat the exercise up to four times. Then turn onto your left side and follow the same sequence on the other side. Repeat up to four times.

exhale   ▶ inhale   exhale   ‖   ▶   ‖

ballet legs *gluteals and adductors*

The combined movements of this exercise stretch and strengthen all the major muscles in the legs and hips. The sequence also challenges your core stability as the legs stretch out. Beginners should only take the leg to 45 degrees and bend the supporting leg. Do not attempt this exercise if you have knee or lower back problems.

● Begin the exercise by lying on your left side with your head resting on your arm. You can use a pillow if this is uncomfortable. Put your other arm in front of your body with the hand flat on the floor.

● With your body in a line through your shoulders, hips, and knees, lift your right leg up, drawing an imaginary line with your toes along you left leg. Beginners should bring their knee to 45 degrees, others to 90 degrees.

● When you reach 45 or 90 degrees, flex the foot and put it down in front of the left leg. Push your right leg up again as far as you can toward your head, and then place it back down again and point both toes together.

● Breathe in and bring your turned out foot toward your knee; then breathe out as you straighten the leg to the ceiling.

inhale ▶ **exhale** ▶ **inhale** **exhale**

intro to 100s *abdominal muscles*

This original Pilates exercise is excellent for strengthening your abdominal muscles. It is important to maintain a neutral spine when the feet are on the floor. Beginners should study the first three images and keep the feet down, using one hand to support the head, before progressing. If you have neck or lower back problems try the beginners version but stop if you feel any strain.

● Start on your back with your knees bent. Have your arms slightly bent and raised level with your ribs. Breathe in and lengthen your spine. Then breathe in and out five times, focusing on hollowing your abdominals.

● Now stretch your arms out beside you, reaching from deep in the pit of your arm as if you were trying to touch a wall on the other side of the room with your fingertips.

● Lift your head up to look at your navel. Make sure you are bending forward from your upper torso and not your neck. Keep the shoulders down, pressing away from your ears so that you stretch the neck.

● When your head is lifted up, raise your right leg up to a 90 degree angle. Keep it bent at the knee with your toes pointed out.

■ inhale and exhale x 5   ‖ inhale   ▶ exhale   ▶ inhale   ▶

● Bring your left leg up to join the right one. Focus on the weight of your stomach as it sinks into your spine, and keep your shoulder blades pressed into the floor.

● Raise both your arms to a 45 degree angle. Maintain your back position on the mat, hollowing your abdominals and not allowing your back to arch.

● You can place a small pillow or rolled towel under your head to give your neck support if you find it too difficult to keep your head lifted throughout this routine.

● Bring your arms back down again, and end by lowering your head and placing the soles of your feet back on the floor again. Remember to keep contracting your lower abs throughout this sequence.

exhale ▶ inhale exhale ‖ ▶ ‖

abdominal muscles and hip flexors

This advanced 100s presents a real challenge to the abdominal muscles. In its most advanced form (end of the image sequence), the muscles at the front of the hip "pay out" as you lower your legs and your core control is tested to the limit. Do not attempt this if you have neck or lower back problems.

● Lie on your back with your hands by your sides. Have your knees at a 90 degree angle to your body with your toes pointing out. Lift your head up and scoop your stomach in. Inhale for five counts and exhale for five counts.

● Reach your hands toward your feet to avoid hunching your shoulders. Raise your right leg up to a 90 degree angle and then bring your left leg up parallel with it. Keep drawing your abs in to support your back.

● Stretch your legs up, then turn your feet out and begin to lower both legs to the floor (advanced level only). Squeeze the buttocks together to provide extra stability for your pelvis.

● Take your legs down to a 45 degree angle and then straighten your feet, pointing your toes away from you. Keep the back of the neck long and make sure you don't protrude your chin.

| ■ inhale and exhale x 5 | ❙❙ inhale ▶ | exhale ▶ | inhale ▶ |

● Now, working from your hip, contract your lower abs and raise your legs into the air again. Keep your shoulders pressing away from your ears to stretch your neck muscles and increase the focus on the abdominals.

● Point your feet and start to lower your legs down again. This time cross your legs over each other as you lower them. If you are straining your back at any point, bend your knees into you chest and relax.

● Keep crossing alternate legs as you bring them down. You can do this movement with flexed feet if it is more comfortable. Keep your pelvis pressed into the mat and do not allow your back to arch.

● Imagine you are holding an orange under your chin to ensure that your neck stays in the correct position. Finish by drawing your knees into your chest and rolling back down to the floor. And relax.

exhale   ▶ inhale   exhale   ‖   ▶   ‖

leg dances

hip flexors and adductors

The dance movement works the lower abdominal muscles
(internal obliques), and the double leg reach works the inner
thighs (adductors) and stretches the hamstrings. Beginners can
keep their toes on the floor, dropping their knees left and right.
Do not attempt this exercise if you have lower back problems.

● Start by sitting upright. Support
yourself with your arms and have your
knees bent with your feet pointed out.
Begin to lean your knees to the right.

● Extend your legs at this angle, with
your head facing in the opposite
direction. Make sure that you keep
your chest lifted (don't let it sink).
Keep your arms as straight as you
can without locking the elbows.

● Take your legs back to the center
again and twist to the other side while
looking in the opposite direction again.
Repeat these extensions between two
and four times on each side.

● Now bend your arms at the elbows
and rest on your forearms. Keep your
neck long. Bend your left knee and
start to lift your right leg up into the
air. Keep your back supported by
engaging your lower abs.

inhale ▶ **exhale** ▶ **inhale** **exhale** ▶ **begin to inhale** ▶

● Turn your leg outward as you lift it up. Keep your toes pointed and then flex your foot when your leg is straight in front of you.

● Slowly lower your leg back down onto the floor again, keeping the leg straight and your foot turned outward. Keep your abdominal muscles pulled in tight for support.

● Breathe in and raise your leg up into the air again with the foot still turned out. Only lift it to a 90 degree angle if this is comfortable (you should not feel any strain in your lower back).

● Repeat the exercise with the other leg. Keep your ribs rolled forward and your legs controlled as you raise and lower them. Finish by uncurling to the relaxation position and breathe deeply.

inhale   ▶   exhale   ▶   inhale   exhale ▶   ‖

advanced mermaid *quadratus lumborum*

This movement is in two parts—a beginners and an advanced Mermaid pose. The sequence stretches and strengthens the muscles of the shoulders, arms, and side of the spine. Beginners should practice the seated pose before progressing. Do not attempt the second part of this exercise if you have neck, shoulder, or wrist problems.

● Begin the sequence sitting upright, with your legs tucked under your body but to one side. Keeping your left hand on the floor, raise your right arm and extend outward so that the arm is parallel with your shoulder.

● Continue to raise your arm and rotate the hand so that the palm is facing inward toward your body. Bend the arm at the elbow to form a gentle curve so that the palm is facing down toward your head.

● With your left hand flat on the floor, lower your body sideway toward the floor. Bend your arm to bring it down and rest on your elbow. Keep your right arm in the same pose throughout so that the palm is now facing down toward the floor.

● Pushing with the left hand, raise your body to sit upright, with your feet still tucked to one side. Once you are sitting upright, lower your right arm and raise your left hand in a smooth flowing movement. Your abdominals should be contracted throughout.

■ **inhale**   **exhale**   ▶   **inhale**   ‖   **exhale**   ▶

● Now bend your body to the right, bringing your right hand down to rest on your right foot. At the same time, face toward the right and raise your left arm. Rotate the palm inward so that the palm extends beyond your head and faces down to the floor.

● Now raise your body back to the center and face forward with both arms extended; then gently lower yourself to the left until your left hand is pressed palm down onto the floor. Slowly extend your legs out from under your body.

● With your head turned down to your left, push your feet into the floor to bring your body upright. Extend your left arm to lock at the elbow and extend your legs out fully. Extend your right arm over your head so that the palm is facing down to the floor.

● Imagine you are suspended at the hips by a sling attached to the ceiling. Hold the pose briefly. Now lower your body back down to the start position. Rest your arms, relax, breathe deeply, and expand your chest. Now do the exercise on the other side.

inhale ▶ exhale inhale ‖ exhale ▶ ‖

half cat and ankle stretch *and tibialis anterior*

The half cat stretches the back and shoulder muscles (spinal extensors and latissimus dorsi).

The knee raise stretches the muscles that run along the front of the lower leg (tibialis anterior).

Do not attempt to press your chest to the floor as shown in the sequence—this is for advanced exercisers only. Do not attempt this exercise if you have knee problems.

● Start by sitting on your heels with your knees tucked under your body and your forehead resting on the floor. Your arms should be fully extended but relaxed. Breathe in and lengthen your spine.

● Lift your head up about six to eight inches. Keep your neck lengthened and then creep forward, lowering your chest to the floor and raising your hips in the air.

● Make sure that your upper legs are vertical and your spine is lengthened as you stretch your upper body.

● Now, scoop your lower abdominals in, tuck your bottom under, and slide back to sit on your heels again. Repeat this exercise slowly and carefully four times.

‖ inhale ▶ exhale ▶ inhale exhale

● After you have finished the four stretches, begin to sit up on your feet. Curl your back and gradually lift your neck up too. Slide your hands back as you raise your chest.

● As you sit up straight, bring your hands to your sides with the fingertips resting on the floor.

● Raise the right knee off the floor a few inches. You can lean slightly back as you do this movement. Put the knee back down again and repeat with the left knee.

● Raise your knees alternately four times each, then bring your hands forward into your lap and rest them on your knees.

inhale ▶ exhale inhale ❚❚ ▶ ❚❚

final release

cat and table legs *pelvic and shoulder girdle stability*

This exercise will strengthen your back muscles and improve spinal flexibility. The "cat" stretches your upper back and shoulders while the leg and arm stretches challenge your core control and hip and shoulder flexibility. If you suffer from knee, shoulder, or wrist problems, approach this exercise with caution.

● Begin this exercise kneeling on all fours keeping the long shallow curves of your spine in the neutral position. Be careful not to put too much pressure on your wrists—if you feel any pain, stop.

● Slowly begin to arch your back up. Curl from the pelvis and lengthen your neck. Keep your arms and legs still to support this movement. Release, straighten your back, and repeat four times.

● Now, lengthen your right leg to its full extent and raise it to a 90 degree angle. Make sure you keep your hips aligned as you do this sequence.

● Bring your leg back down again. Repeat the exercise using the other leg. Keep looking down at the floor and don't let your head and neck drop. Only lift your leg as high as you can keep your pelvis square.

■ inhale   exhale   ‖   inhale   exhale   ▶   inhale   ▶

● Keeping your pelvis square, your spine lengthened and your shoulders relaxed, lift the right arm forward toward a 90 degree angle. Beginners should keep the arm in a low "salute."

● Bring the arm slowly down again and repeat this exercise with the other arm. Make sure you don't twist from the hips. Keep your neck long, your back flat and your lower abdominals pulled into your spine.

● Now, combine the arm and leg movements. Begin with your left leg and right arm, and raise them both slowly. Keep your shoulders down and concentrate on lengthening the spine and pulling in the lower abdominals.

● Lower your arms and legs to the floor again, and then repeat this movement with your right leg and left arm.

exhale ▶ inhale ‖ exhale inhale ‖ exhale inhale ‖ exhale

advanced table legs *shoulder girdle stability*

This exercise is named the "table," as this image helps remind you to keep your hips and shoulders horizontal as you work through the stretch. The leg and arm reach works your hip and shoulder muscles, and tests your balance and core control. Do not attempt this exercise if you have knee, shoulder, or lower back problems.

● Kneel forward and place your hands under your shoulders with your fingers facing forward. Have your back straight, your knees at a right angle to your body, and look down at the floor. Breathe in and lengthen the spine.

● Contract your lower abdominals and extend your left leg and right arm at the same time. If you have a strong center (a balance of good abdominals and back muscles) you can continue to stretch your limbs a little further.

● Breathe in and then on a breath out, bring your leg and arm down again, and start to bend your knee in toward your body. Keep your neck lengthened and your supporting leg and arm steady.

● Taking care not to twist your body as you move your leg, start to bend your head in toward your knee. Make sure your shoulders are not hunched and that your lower abdominals keep working.

 ⏸ **exhale**   ▶   **inhale**   **exhale**   **inhale**   ▶

● Bring your knee up to your chin and your right elbow bent into the side of your body. Keep your stomach hollowed throughout this sequence and your shoulders down.

● Start to extend your right arm and your left leg again. Remember that most people stop this movement when their limbs are horizontal. Only attempt to raise your limbs higher if you are at an advanced level.

● Hold the pose briefly and then take your arm and leg back down toward your torso again.

● Finish this part of the exercise on all fours as you did at the beginning. Then repeat the sequence on the other side, stretching the left arm and the right leg.

begin to exhale ▶ exhale inhale ‖ ▶ ‖

shoulder brace with stretch band

shoulder girdle and latissimus dorsi

This exercise can help increase the mobility of the shoulder joint by stretching key muscles in the shoulder girdle. Beginners should keep the arm movements small at first. Do not attempt this exercise if you have shoulder or neck problems.

● Stand up straight with your hands at hip height and holding the stretch band in front of you. Breathe in and contract your lower abdominals imagining you are lengthening your spine from the top of your head.

● Bring the band up in front of you. Keep your elbows slightly bent and lift the band up over your head.

● Stretch as you bring your arms over your head and down behind your back toward your buttocks. Keep your shoulders down and your neck relaxed.

● Try to lengthen right up out of your waist as you bring the band down again in front of you.

● Repeat this action, bringing the band up over your head. When your arms are directly above your head, bend both your elbows.

● Lower the band behind your back and move your arms down so they are at a right angle to your body. When you reach shoulder level, extend them fully if this is comfortable.

● Keeping your arms straight, raise your arms slowly back over your head again, bring them down in front of you, and then relax. Repeat up to eight times.

inhale   ▶   **begin to exhale**   **exhale**   ‖   ▶   ‖

side stretch and twist with pole

This exercise stretches key muscles in your upper back and spine (latissimus dorsi and quadratus lumborum), and the oblique abdominals. Beginners should practice sitting on a chair as this keeps the pelvis stable. If you have back or shoulder problems, try the sitting version without the pole. Stop if you feel any discomfort.

● Begin standing up with your arms wrapped over the pole (you can use a broom handle), holding it with a firm grip. Breathe in, lengthen the spine, and contract your lower abdominals.

● Dip over to your right-hand side as far as you can. Turn your head to look toward your right hand. Remember to keep your body facing forward and feel the stretch along your side. Only go as far as is comfortable.

● Come back up again so your body is straight and your arms are at right angles. Dip over to your left side. Try to get your arms vertical, but do not strain at all or allow your lower abdominals to bulge or "dome".

● Return to your starting position and as you breathe out, begin to twist around to the right. Turn your head to follow your arm. Keep your shoulders down, your neck relaxed, and your spine lengthened.

● Keep your hips straight as you twist. You should feel the stretch in your waist. Twist around as far as is comfortable and then return to the center. Think of working your abdominals and back muscles together.

● Now twist your upper body around to the left. Remember to keep your lower body stable and only twist from the waist. Keep your knees soft and your feet about hip width apart.

● Twist your waist around as far as is comfortable, take a breath in, and then return to the center. Repeat this whole sequence up to five times.

inhale   exhale   ▶ inhale   exhale   ‖   ▶   ‖

lateral raise with arm weights
rhomboids, latissimus and deltoids

This exercise will strengthen your back and shoulder muscles (rhomboids, latissimus dorsi, trapezius, and deltoids). Beginners should practice sitting on a chair leaning forward to a 30 degree angle. If you have shoulder or back problems try the sitting version, but stop if you feel any discomfort.

● Begin standing up. Bend over at the waist so your body is at a 90 degree angle. Imagine your back is as flat as a table with your shoulders open and not hunched. Have your arms loose and palms facing back.

● Keep your feet parallel and bend the elbows up as far as you can. Make sure your knees are bent slightly and that your hands keep facing down.

● Lower your arms back down again, making sure your head remains aligned with your spine and does not hang forward at all. Repeat this exercise. Keep your lower abdominals pulled in to support your back.

● Now bend your elbows out to the sides so that they are parallel to your shoulders, or slightly higher, and repeat. Make sure this is a slow and controlled movement.

 inhale   exhale   ▶ inhale   exhale ▶ inhale   ▶

● Breathe out as you bring your arms together. Now, inhale and simultaneously extend your right arm straight out in front of you and the other arm straight behind you.

● Be careful not to throw your arms forward or back. All movements should be slow and controlled with the deeper abdominal muscles pulling in around the waist throughout the exercise.

● Exhale and bring your arms back in front of you again. Keep the shoulders down and your abdomen engaged. If your back hurts at any point during this exercise, stop immediately.

● Inhale as you repeat the sequence with the opposite arm leading. Make sure your extended arms are parallel to your body. Repeat up to eight times.

exhale   **inhale** ▶   **begin to exhale**   ▶   **exhale**   ▶   **inhale**

roll ups with pole abdominals, hip flexors and vertbrae

The roll-up is an original Pilates exercise that stretches all the muscles along the back of your body, articulates the spine, and strengthens your abdominals which can help flatten the stomach. The pole is used to help keep your arms parallel and shoulders level. Beginners should only roll-up half way, keeping the knees bent. Do not do this exercise if you have lower back or shoulder problems.

● Lie on your back and lengthen your body. Your arms should be straight behind your head. Have your palms facing up and your feet flexed. Hollow your lower abdominals by pulling them into your spine.

● Squeeze your buttocks tightly and press the back of your upper inner thighs together. Begin to raise your arms straight up, bringing your head, neck, and back up, too. Inhale as you begin to roll up and forward.

● Be careful not to let your legs lift off the mat as you roll up. Fold all the way forward as far as you can, then breathe out as you stretch forward from the hips while keeping your stomach pulled back into your spine.

● Start to roll down by squeezing your buttocks together and slightly tucking your tailbone underneath you. Breathe in as you begin pulling your stomach into your spine again.

■ inhale   inhale ▶   exhale ▶   inhale ▶

● Breathe out as you bend your knees and begin to roll back down. Feel each vertebra pressing into the floor as you descend slowly and carefully, keeping your lower abdominals drawn in toward them.

● Keep squeezing the back of your upper inner thighs together for stability, and keep your chin tucked into your chest so you are not pulling from the neck.

● Concentrate on lengthening the spine as you do this exercise. Keep the lower body still, and focus on the spinal muscles.

● When the back of your shoulders touch the floor, lower your head and bring your arms over it. Stretch your body out fully, then repeat the exercise between four and eight times.

begin to exhale ▶ **exhale** ▶ **exhale** ▶ **inhale**

teaser abdominals and hip flexors

This original Pilates exercise is a demanding workout for the abdominals and hip muscles. It also challenges your core control and your balance as you coordinate arms and legs. Beginners can try the version shown up to one leg raise. Do not attempt this exercise if you have lower back or neck problems.

● Start this exercise lying on your back with your arms straight out above your head. Hollow your lower abdominals in toward the spine and press your lower back gently into the mat without tucking.

● Breathe in and lengthen the spine. Breathe out and straighten your right leg up to a 45 degree angle. Press the knees together. Hold your leg in this position and squeeze your buttocks and inner thighs together tightly.

● Now, raise your arms above your head and allow your head and upper body to begin to lift from the floor, too. Reach your hands toward your outstretched toes, and lift out of your waist as you breathe in.

● As you breathe out, begin to roll your spine slowly back down on the floor. Keep your right leg up in the air, and stretch your arms back over your head. Beginners can roll back down and repeat with the other leg.

inhale   II   exhale   inhale   ▶   exhale   ▶

● Now, bring the left leg up to join the other leg. Keep your toes pointed and make sure you maintain a flat and stable back.

● Lower your legs to a 45 degree angle. Inhale, bring your arms over your head and reach toward your toes, creating a V shape. Balancing on your tailbone, hold this pose with your abdominals pulled into your spine.

● Breathe out as you begin rolling your spine back down onto the floor again. Squeeze your buttocks to help keep your pelvis stable and support the weight of your legs.

● When your head touches the floor, stretch your arms out over your head again and bend your knees. Repeat this whole sequence up to five times as your stamina and strength improves.

exhale ▶ inhale ‖ exhale ▶ inhale ■

advanced
boomerang *abdominals and hip flexors*

The boomerang (an original Pilates exercise) is one of the most comprehensive you can do as it stretches and strengthens all the major muscle groups in your body. It is a particularly good workout for the abdominals and hip flexors, develops suppleness in your spine, legs and shoulders, and challenges your balance. Avoid this exercise if you suffer from neck, back, or shoulder problems

● Breathe in and straighten your spine. Sit tall with your legs straight out in front of you, your arms by your sides and your neck and shoulders relaxed.

● Bend your knees up to your body and start to roll back, extending your legs as you do, so they are straight. Slide your arms down onto the floor and use your palms to help push your legs up and back.

● Breathe in and roll back until your legs are over your head. Be careful not to roll onto your neck. Remember to keep your lower abdominals contracted.

● Now, reverse the action and roll forward, keeping your legs straight. Make sure your arms are straight and parallel to your shoulders. Draw your abdominals toward your spine to hold your center.

| inhale | ▶ | exhale | ▶ | inhale | ▶ | begin to exhale | ▶ |

● Keep rolling forward until you are sitting up tall. Extend your arms out to the sides of your body at a 45 degree angle.

● Breathe out and begin to roll forward, bending from the waist. Move your arms out behind you, stretching them away from your torso as you bend.

● Slowly lean forward as far as you can go. Circle your arms forward and aim to reach your toes so your nose is on your knees in a deep bow. Let your neck relax as you stretch forward.

● Contract your lower abdominals and roll back up to the starting position. Keep your legs straight with your toes pointed, and finish with your arms by your sides and sitting up straight. Repeat up to five times.

| exhale | ▶ | exhale | ▶ | inhale | ❚❚ | exhale | inhale | exhale |

chalk circles *pectoralis major*

This exercise mobilizes the spine and stretches your pectoral muscles, helping to release tension in your shoulders and upper back. It is a gentle exercise, but you should still approach it carefully if you have any spinal problems. You can repeat this exercise up to 10 times.

● Start by lying on your right side with your legs bent at the knee at a 90 degree angle to your body. Put your hands together with your arms straight out in front of you. If your neck hurts, place a pillow under it.

● Breathe out and begin to slowly move your left arm along the floor toward the top of your head.

● Stretch your arm over your head, keeping your fingers on the floor if possible. Imagine you are drawing a wide circle with a piece of chalk as you circle your arm over to the other side of your head.

● Breathe out as you open your chest and turn your head toward your left arm, relaxing as best as you can. Hold this position and then take a deep breath in visualizing your chest opening and stretching.

■ inhale ‖ exhale ▶ inhale ▶ exhale ‖ inhale

● Breathe out, tighten your stomach muscles, and then start to move your left arm in a circle down toward your buttocks. Bend your elbow if this is more comfortable.

● Stretch your arm out and move your palm down, as you pass your hip—this will give your neck a good stretch. Keep your abdominal muscles engaged to support your back.

● Breathe in as you place your hands together to complete the circle. Keep your knees at a 90 degree angle at all times to avoid straining your lower back.

● Repeat this exercise four times, then lie on your left side and follow the same circular movement with your right arm.

exhale   ▶ exhale   inhale   ❚❚   ▶   ❚❚

index